BLUE SKY

WHITE CLOUDS

A Book for Memory-Challenged Adults

ELIEZER SOBEL

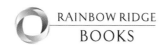

RAINBOW RIDGE
BOOKS

Cover and interior design by Frame 25 Productions
Cover photo © Triff c/o Shutterstock.com

Published by:
Rainbow Ridge Books, LLC
140 Rainbow Ridge Road
Faber, Virginia 22938
434-361-1723

If you are unable to order this book from your local
bookseller, you may order directly from the distributor.

Square One Publishers, Inc.
115 Herricks Road
Garden City Park, NY 11040
Phone: (516) 535-2010
Fax: (516) 535-2014
Toll-free: 877-900-BOOK

Visit the author at:
www.eliezersobel.com

Library of Congress Cataloging-in-Publication Data applied for.

ISBN 978-1-937907-07-5

10 9 8 7 6 5 4 3 2

Printed on acid-free recycled paper in the United States of America

For my beloved Mom

Fairly early on in the progression of my mother's Alzheimer's Disease, she could no longer follow stories or read books. Within a short time, she lost the ability to retain the meaning of even two consecutive sentences. Eventually she was robbed of nearly all ordinary language and

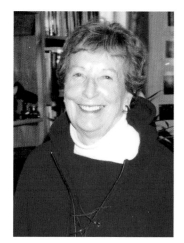

speaking skills, though she continues even now to be quite engaging and talkative, using nonsense words that she makes up as she goes along.

"The mingleman is faleetered nosty?" she will ask me, and I'll reply, "Yes, he is," and we will converse like this for quite a long time. Periodically, out of the blue, some real English will suddenly surprise all of us: "I'm glad I had you," she said to me one day, and I was stunned, for ordinarily she is unaware that she has been married 66 years and has two grown children. Yet she always seems to know and love my brother and me, *whoever* we are!

One day a few years ago I had an astounding revelation: Mom was thumbing through a magazine, looking at the pictures, and I heard her reciting the big print aloud. *My mother can still read,* I realized. Maybe not a book; maybe not a paragraph, or even a full sentence; but she could still read individual words and short phrases.

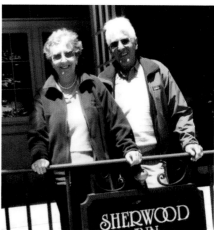

I tried in vain to find an "adult picture book" for someone like her. Something simple, with high quality photos of familiar objects, people and nature, with short, easy-to-read captions. A book in which each page would be complete unto itself, requiring no power of recall.

What you're holding in your hands is the result. I hope and pray that it will provide Alzheimer's patients and other memory-challenged adults, along with their loved ones and caregivers, the opportunity to spend much quality, quiet time together, looking through *Blue Sky, White Clouds* and reading it aloud.

As I write this, my mother, Manya Sobel, has had Alzheimer's disease for nearly ten years, and remains at home under the loving and devoted, constant care of my father, Max Sobel. May they and the millions of people in a similar position be blessed to live peacefully with this very difficult and challenging illness.

Photo Credits:

MORTON D. RICH
Welcoming Finch – Page 1
Dancing in Romania – Page 4
Blue Bicycle – Page 18
www.zazenphoto.smugmug.com

HAL SCHNEE
Charlie Louvin – Page 21
www.astillmind.net

TIM STEPHENSON
In the Pink – Page 6
En Tango – Page 8
www.trinitystreet.com

Shutterstock.com and Istockphoto.com

Deep Appreciation and Gratitude to:

Mort Rich, my dear friend and 9th grade English teacher, for his fabulous photos and hours of tireless effort in support of this project;
Lawrence J. Reynolds, for showing up in my life out of nowhere, making me compose country music, shoot a pistol, and acting like I'm a writer;
Bob Friedman of Rainbow Ridge Books for taking a spontaneous leap of faith;
Jonathan Friedman, our gifted and multi-talented graphic designer;
Hal Schnee and Tim Stephenson for their generous spirit in contributing photos to the book;
and to my "other eyes," my wonderful, one-of-a-kind wife, Shari Cordon.

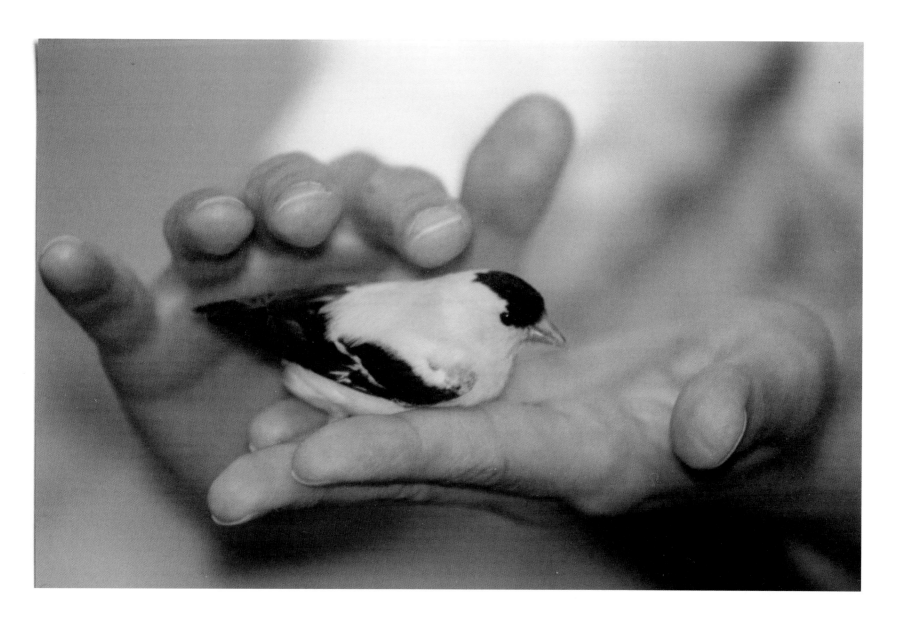

A tiny yellow bird.

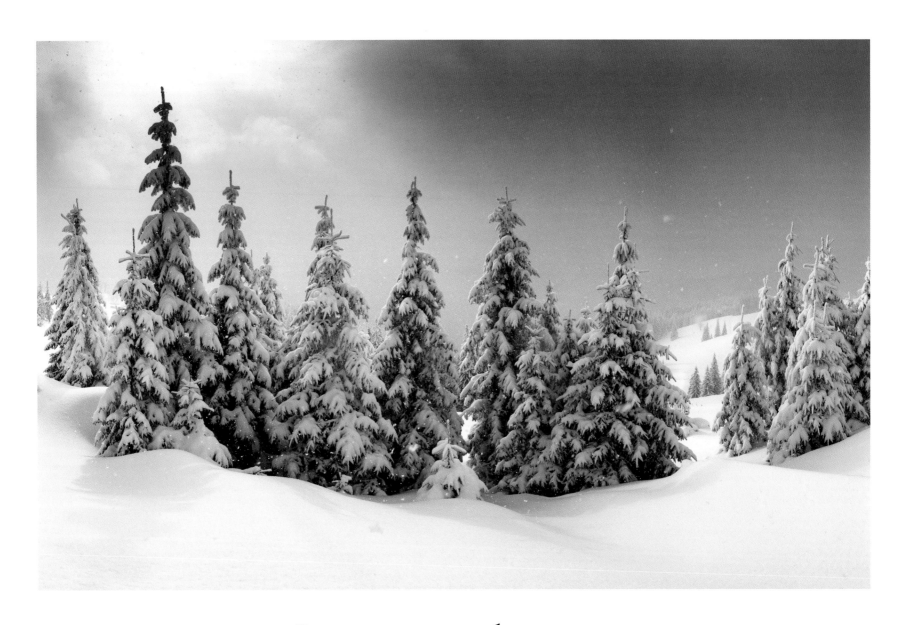

Snow covers the trees.

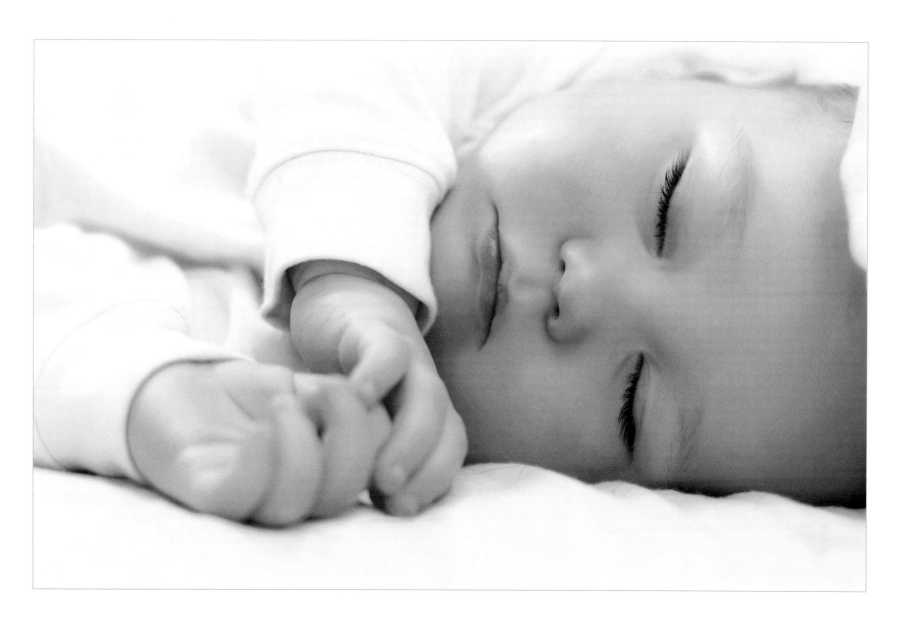

The baby is fast asleep.

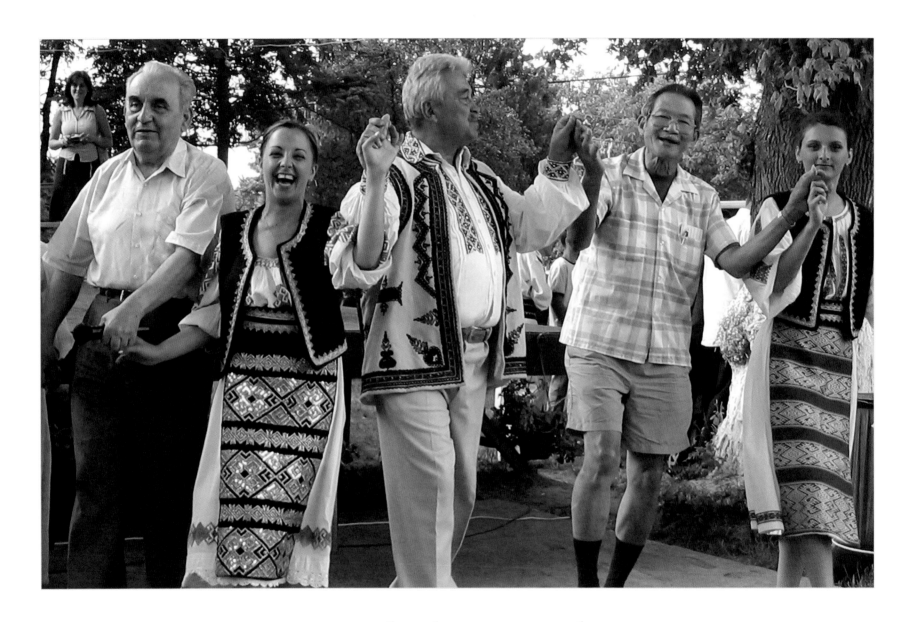

Happy people dance on the street.

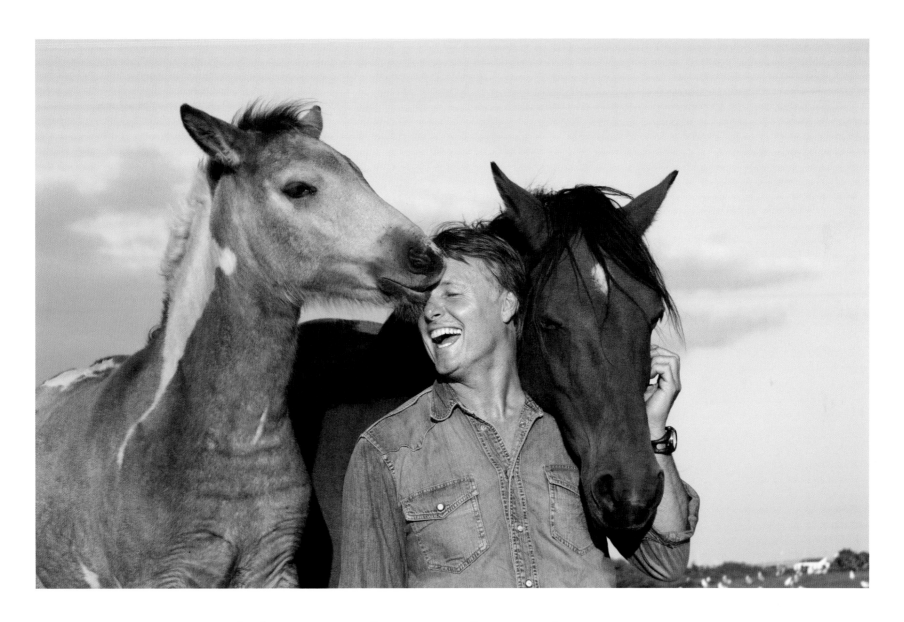

The two horses love the man.

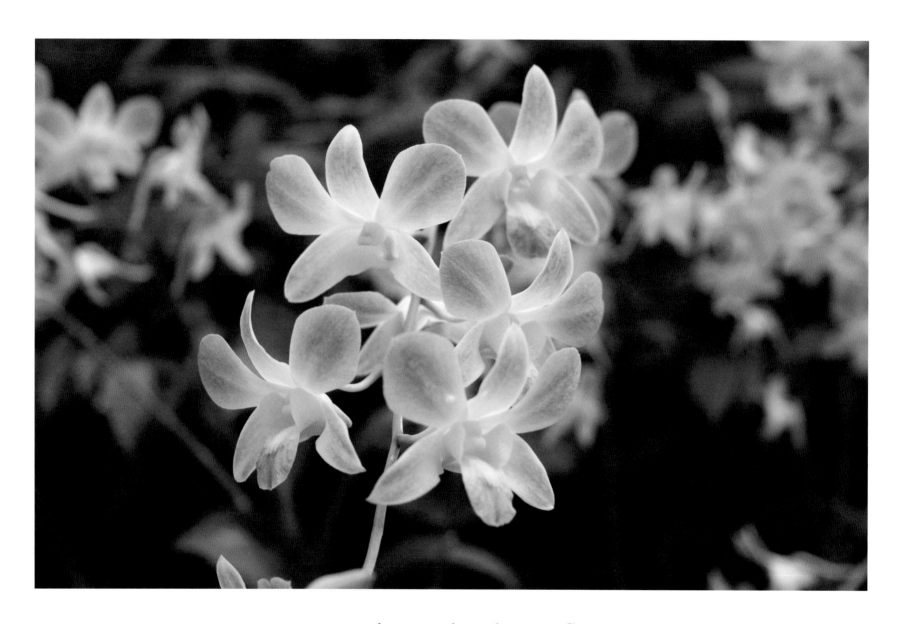

Pretty pink and white flowers.

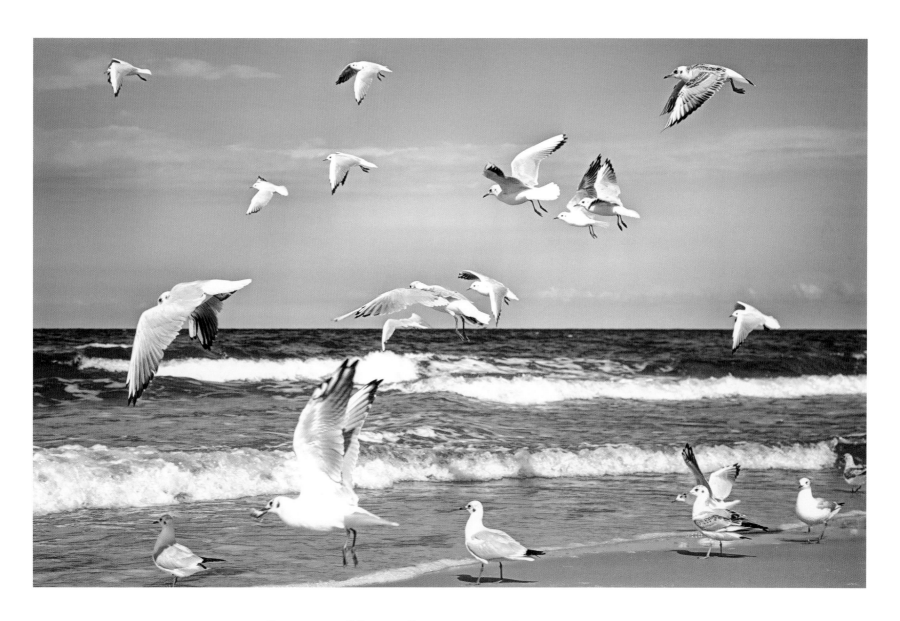

Seagulls play in the water.

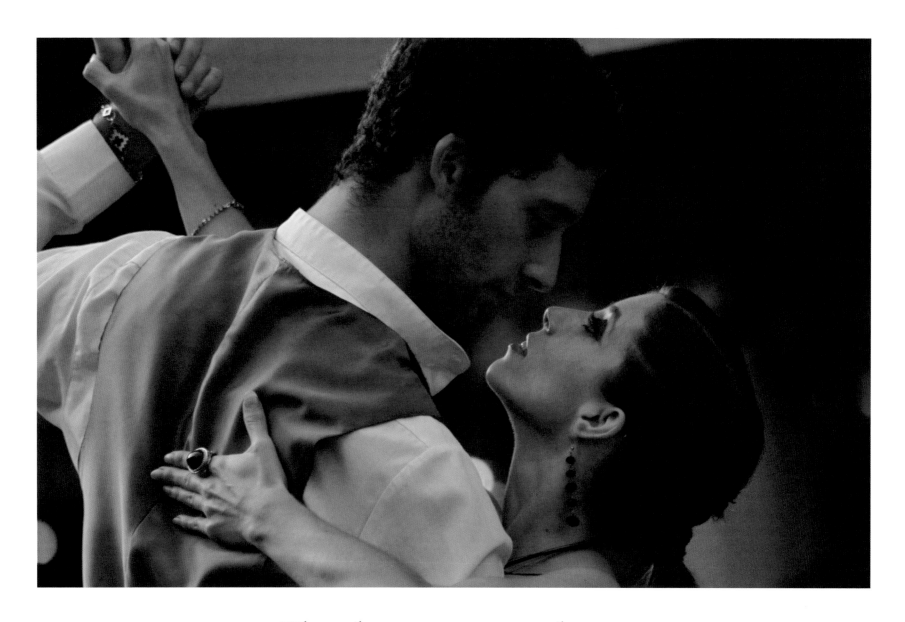

The dancers are in love.

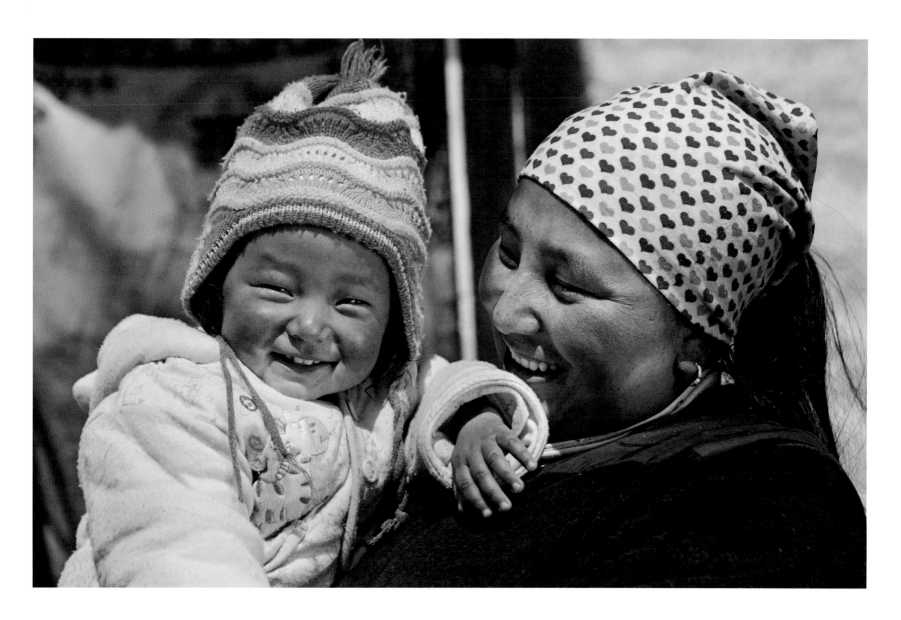

The mother and child are laughing.

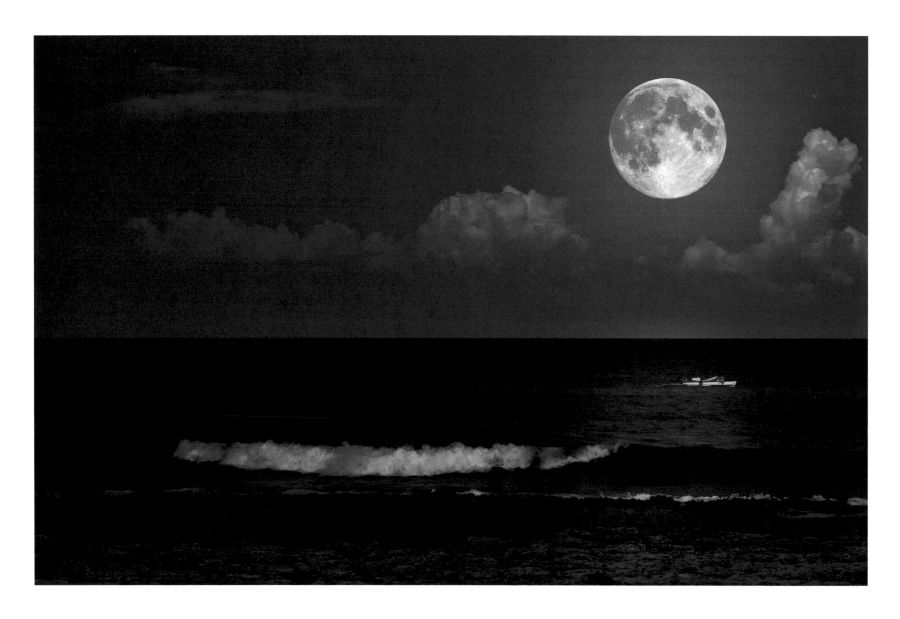

The moon is full tonight.

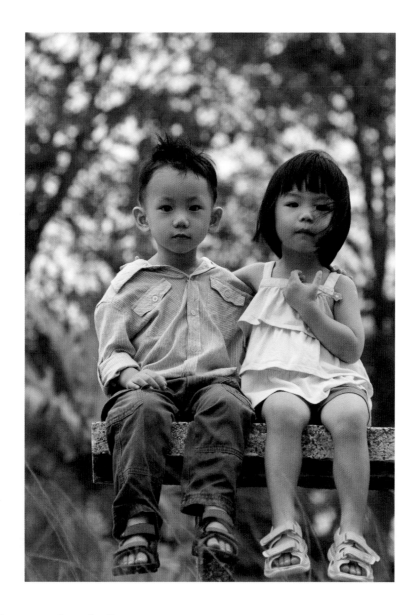

The children are sitting outside.

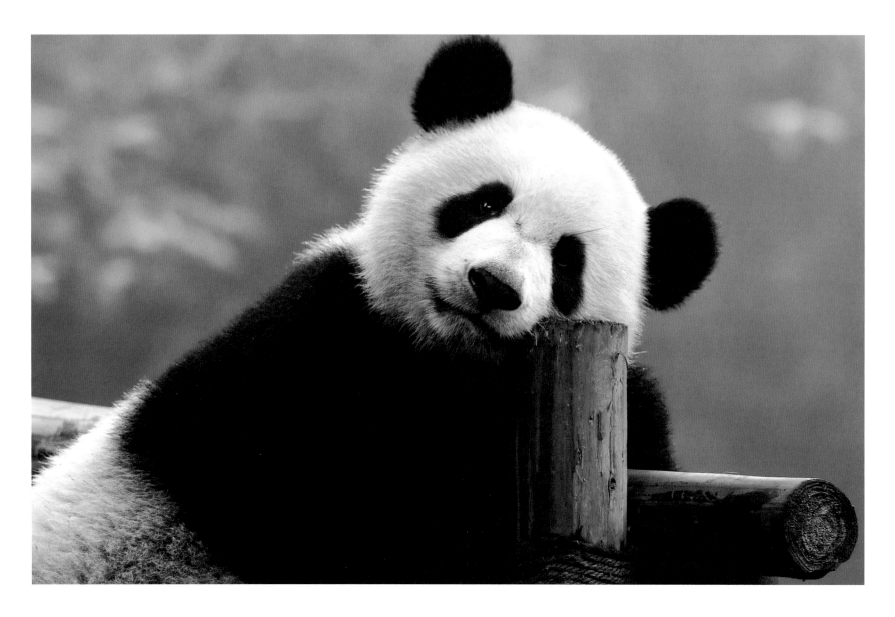

The panda bear is resting.

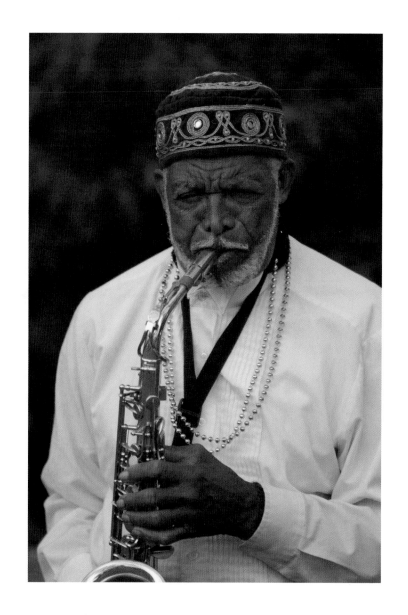

He loves to make music!

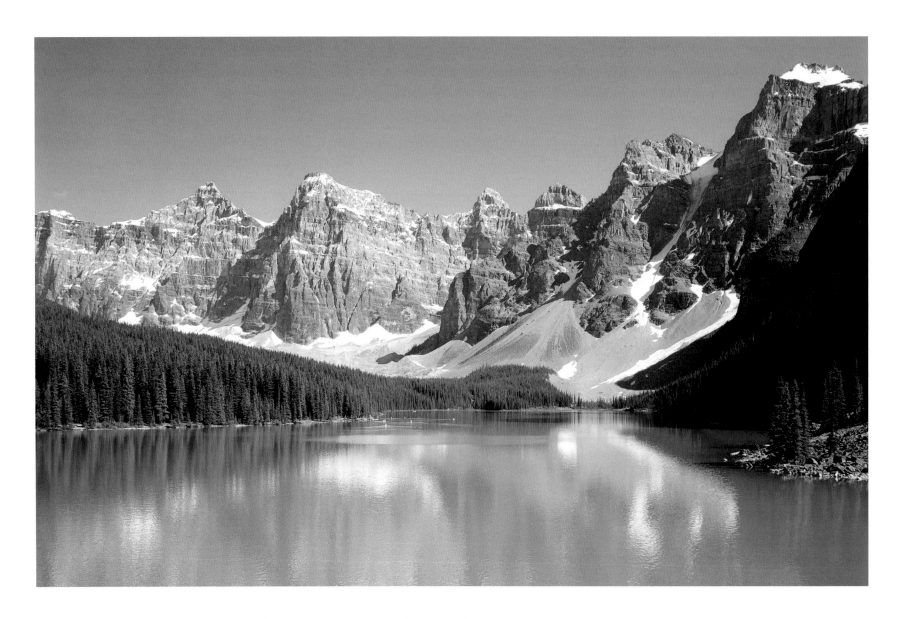

A blue lake by the mountains.

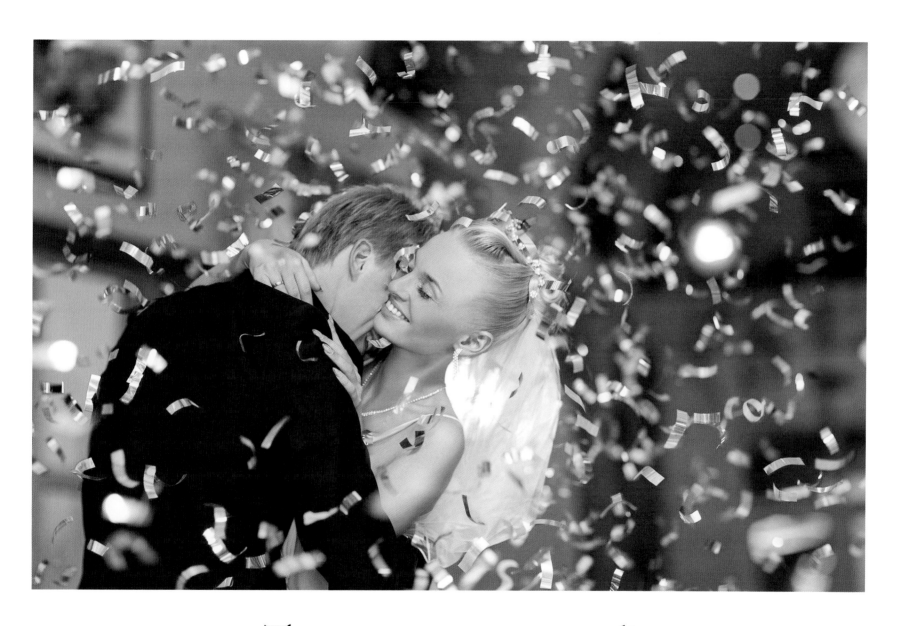

They are getting married!

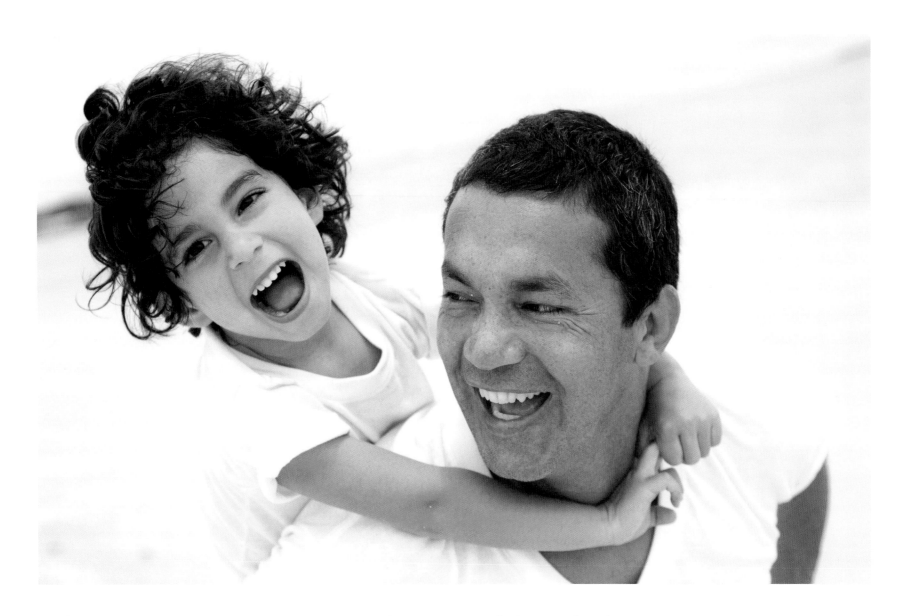

A young boy and his father.

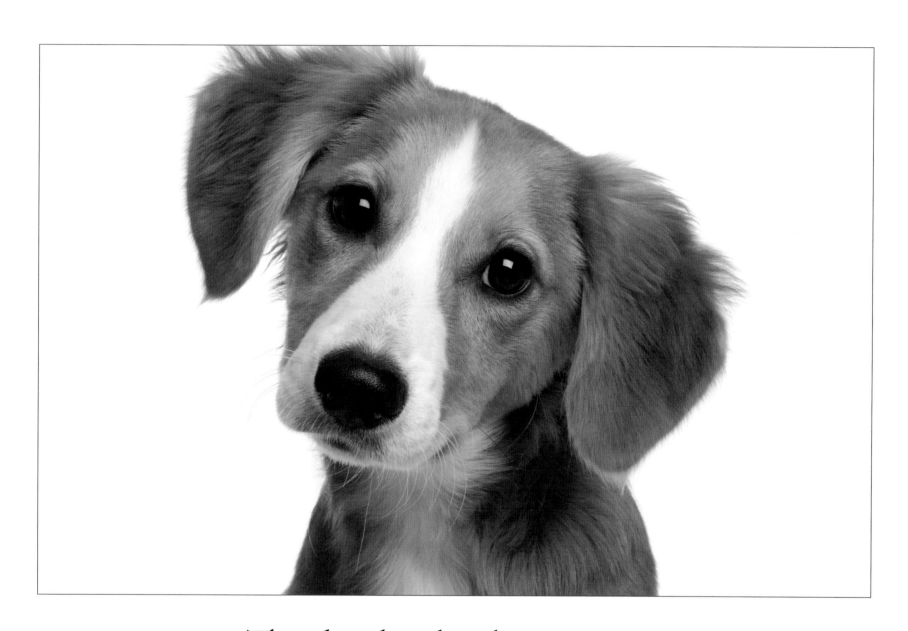

The dog has big brown eyes.

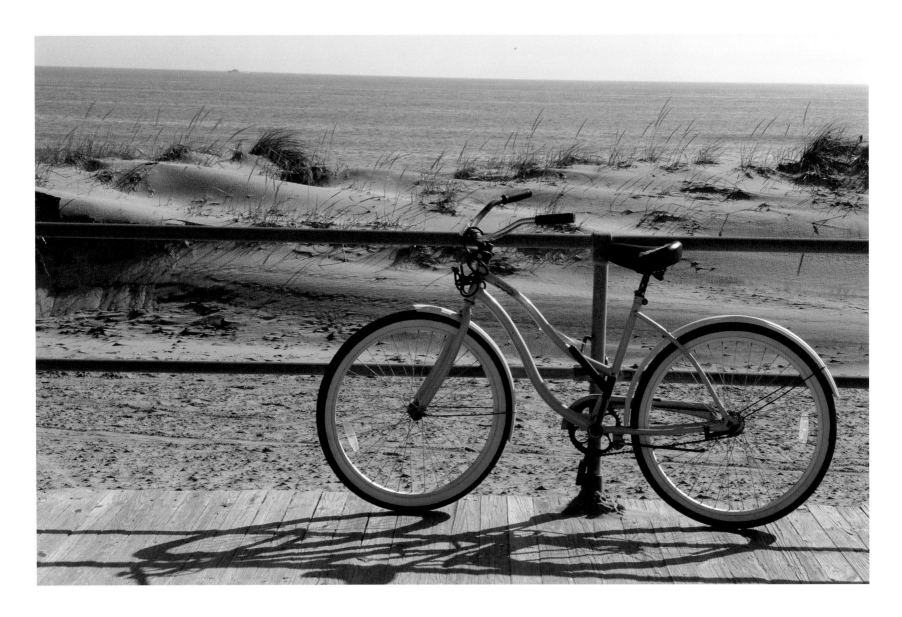

A blue bicycle by the beach.

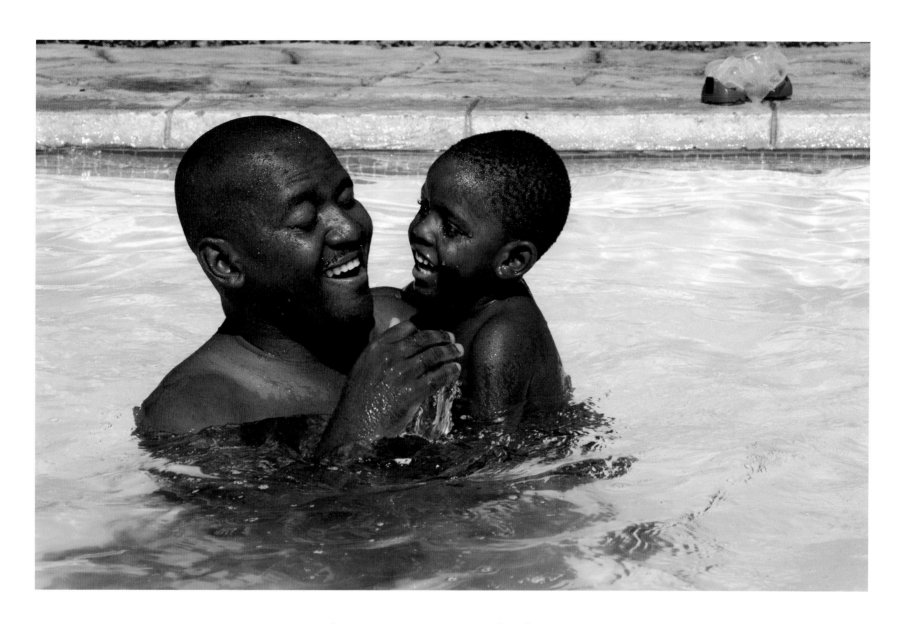

Dad swims with his son.

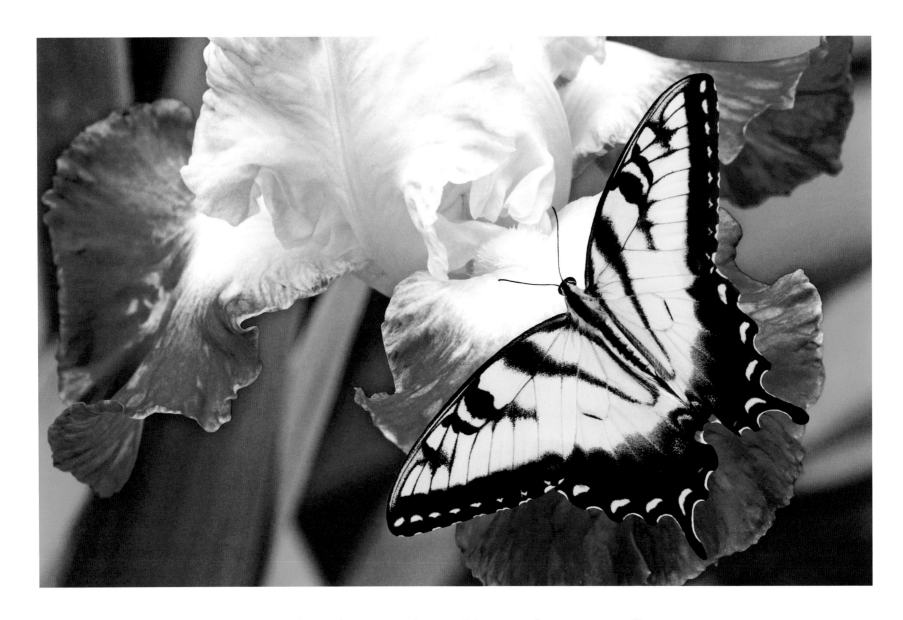

A black and yellow butterfly.

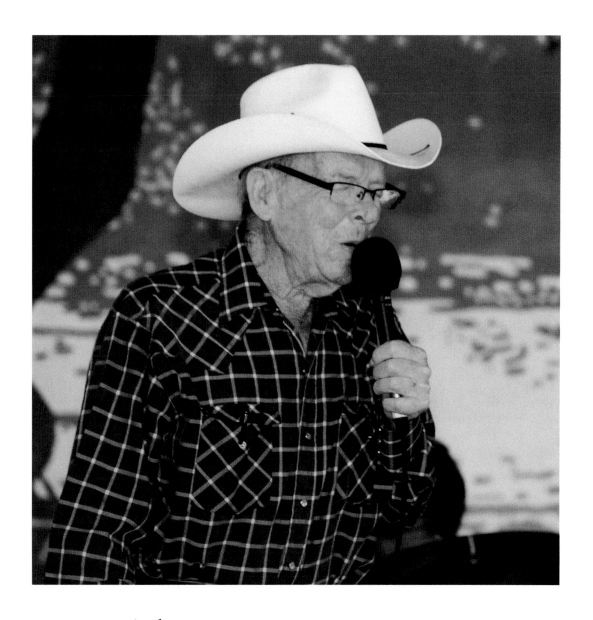

The man sings a song.

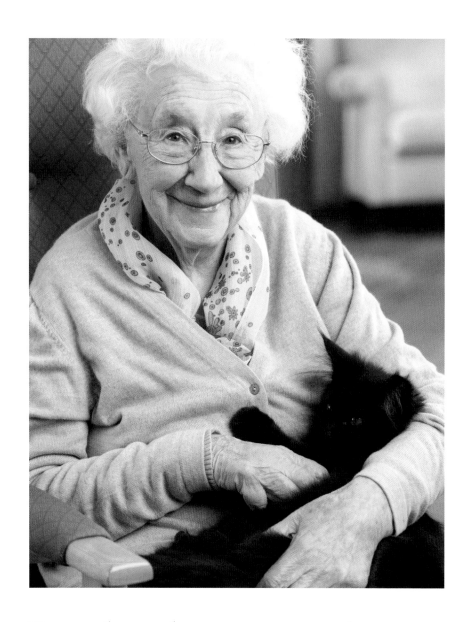

Grandma loves to pet her cat.

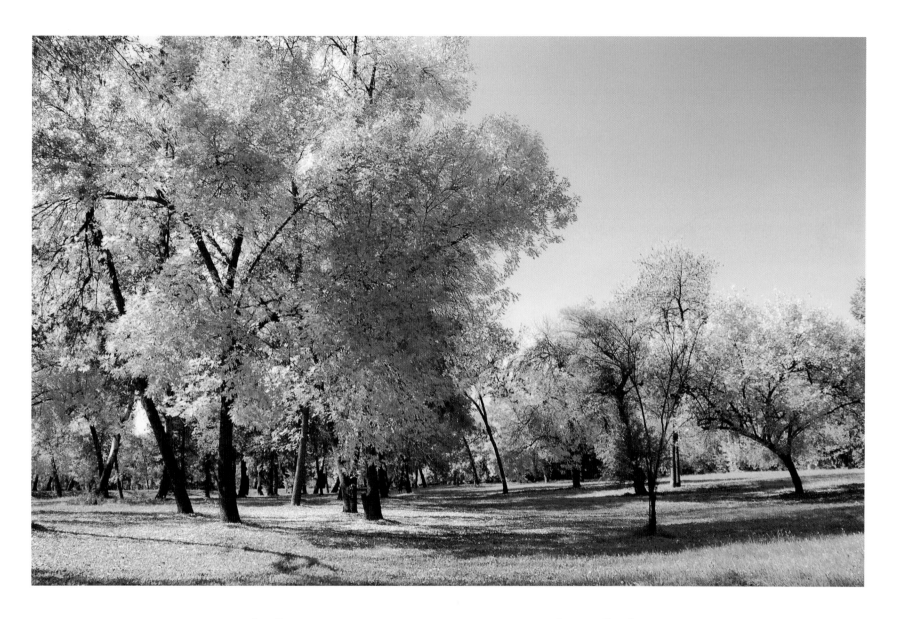

The trees are very colorful.

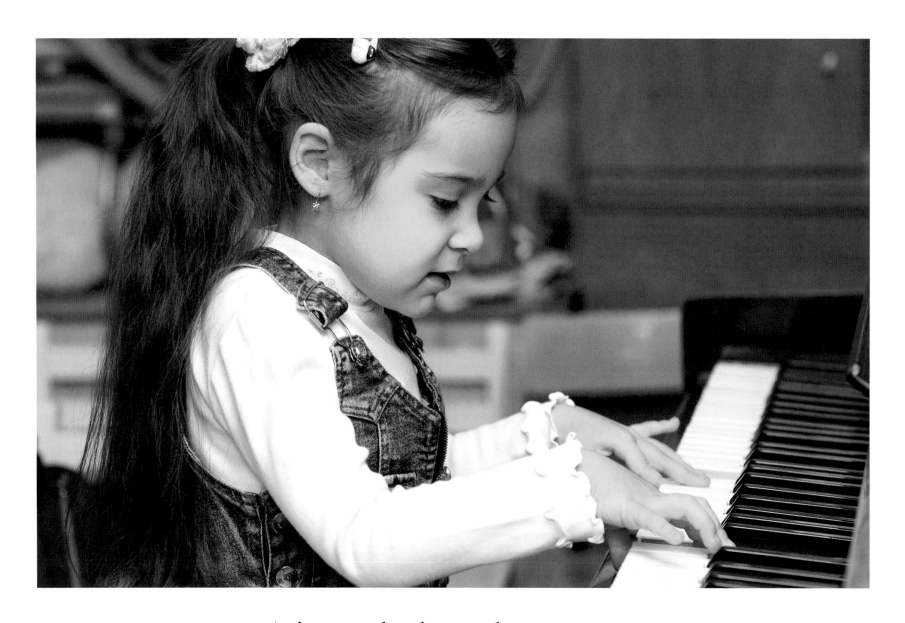

The girl plays the piano.

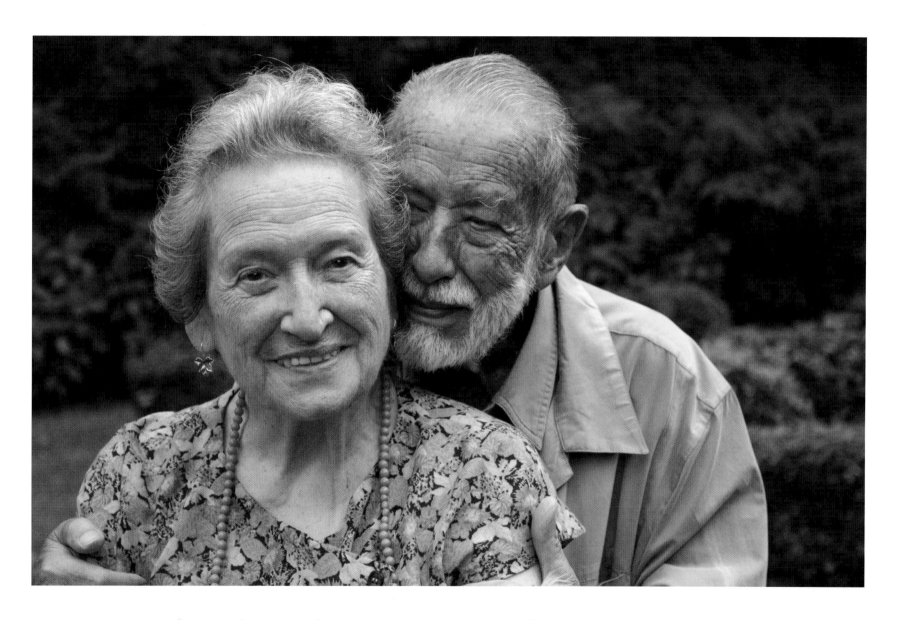

They have been married for many years.

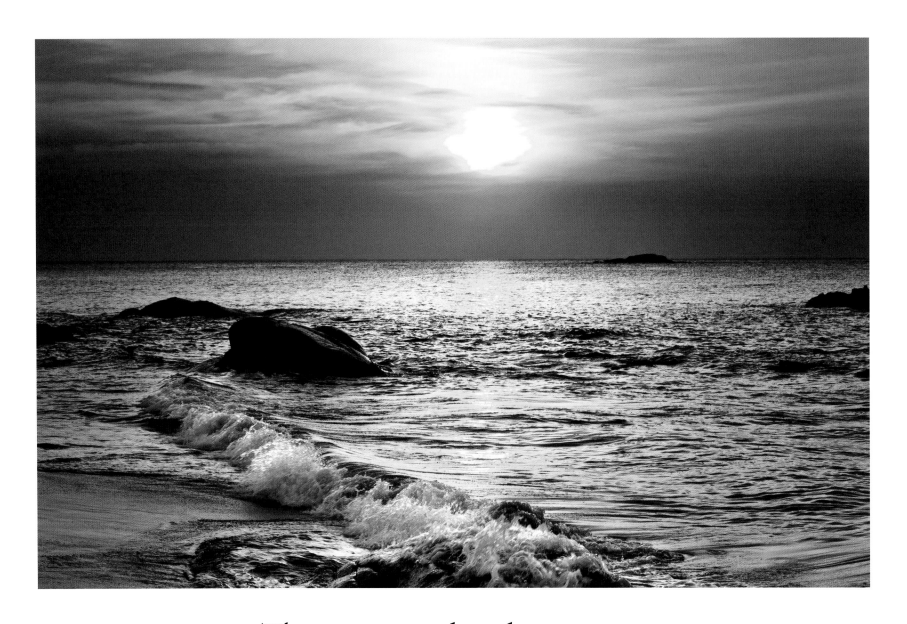

The sun sets by the ocean.

About the Author

ELIEZER SOBEL is the author of *Minyan: Ten Jewish Men in a World That is Heartbroken* (University of Tennessee Press, 2004), selected by National Book Award winner John Casey as the winner of the prestigious Peter Taylor Prize For the Novel; a memoir, *The 99th Monkey: A Spiritual Journalist's Misadventures with Gurus, Messiahs, Sex, Psychedelics and Other Consciousness-Raising Experiments* (Santa Monica Press, 2008); and *Wild Heart Dancing: A Personal One-Day Quest to Liberate the Artist and Lover Within* (Simon & Schuster/Fireside, 1994).

He is also the former publisher and editor of the *Wild Heart Journal* and *The New Sun* magazine, and his blogs regularly appear online on *The Huffington Post* and *Psychology Today*. His articles, short stories, and poetry have appeared in the *Village Voice, Yoga Journal, Tikkun, Quest, New Age Journal, Inner Directions, Epoch, The Widower, Hook, Mudfish, The Minetta Review, Magical Blend, Zeek,* and the *Journal of Pastoral Care*, and many online sites, including *Reality Sandwich, Serene Ambition, Killing the Buddha,* and numerous others.

Sobel has led intensive creativity workshops and retreats around the United States, at Esalen Institute in Big Sur, California, the Open Center in New York City, the Isabella Freedman Jewish Retreat Center in Connecticut, the Lama Foundation in New Mexico, and similar venues.

He has been a hospital chaplain and a nursing home volunteer, a teacher of the 5Rhythms™ Movement Practice, a high school teacher, and the music director for several children's theater companies, and has recently performed in *Narrow Bridge,* an original two-man show about being raised in the shadow of the Holocaust. He lives in Richmond, Virginia with his wife, Shari Cordon.

Related Titles

If you enjoyed *Blue Sky, White Clouds*, look for more titles to come in the series.
You may also enjoy these other Rainbow Ridge titles:

Difficult People: A Gateway to Enlightenment by Lisette Larkins

Thank Your Wicked Parents by Richard Bach

*Consciousness: Bridging the Gap Between Conventional Science
and the New Super Science of Quantum Mechanics* by Eva Herr

Messiah's Handbook: Reminders for the Advanced Soul by Richard Bach

Read more about them at *www.rainbowridgebooks.com*

———————————————

Rainbow Ridge Books is distributed by Square One Publishers in Garden City Park, New York.

To contact authors and editors, peruse our titles,
and see submission guidelines, please visit our website at:

www.rainbowridgebooks.com

For orders and catalogs, please call toll-free:
(877) 900-BOOK